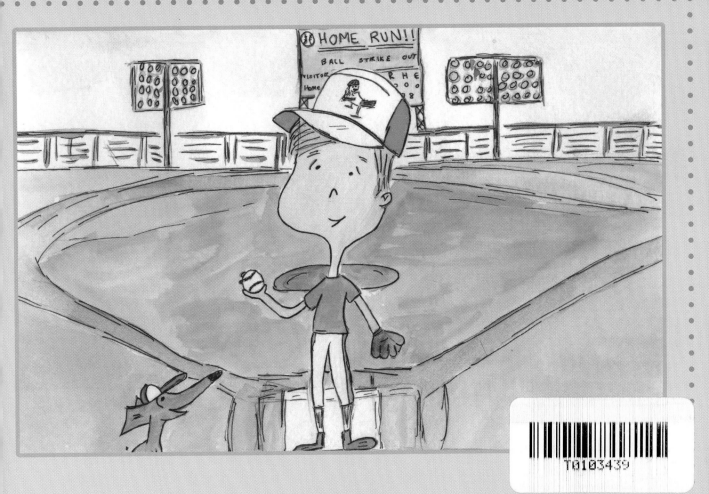

Hi there!

I heard you have a single ventricle.

Welcome to the club!

I was born with only one ventricle as well.

Don't worry. I will tell you all about it!

1

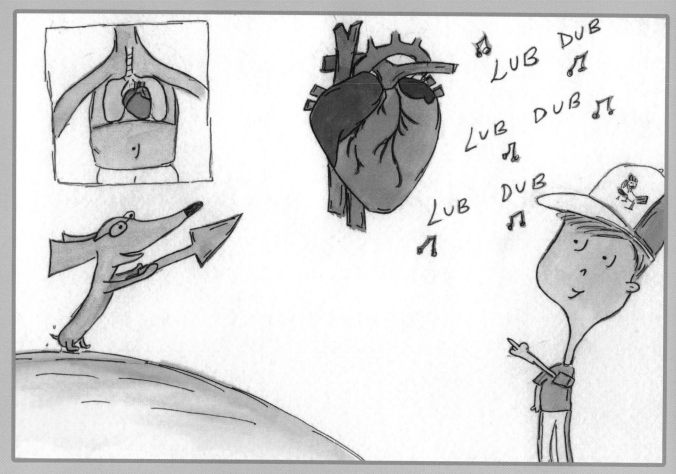

So first, let's talk about hearts. Everybody has a heart.
It sits up in your chest. It is a strong muscle with two
pumping chambers that sends blood all around your body.
From your head to your toes!
It beats – LUB DUB LUB DUB LUB DUB.
Put your hand on your chest. You can even feel it!

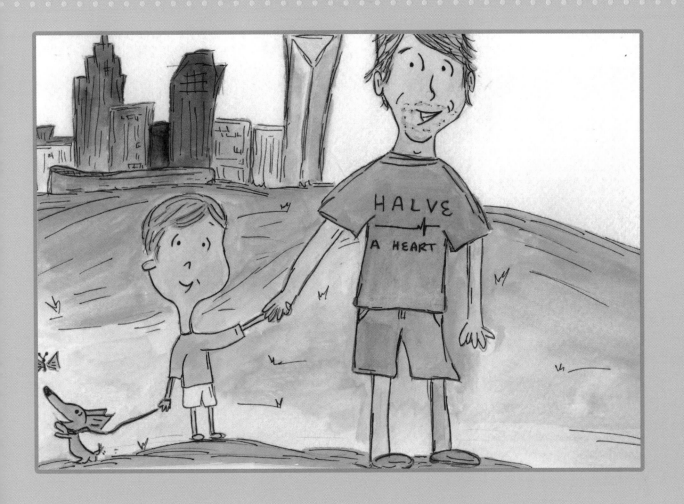

Now our hearts are a little different
because we were born with a single ventricle
— one pumping chamber instead of two.
What does that mean?

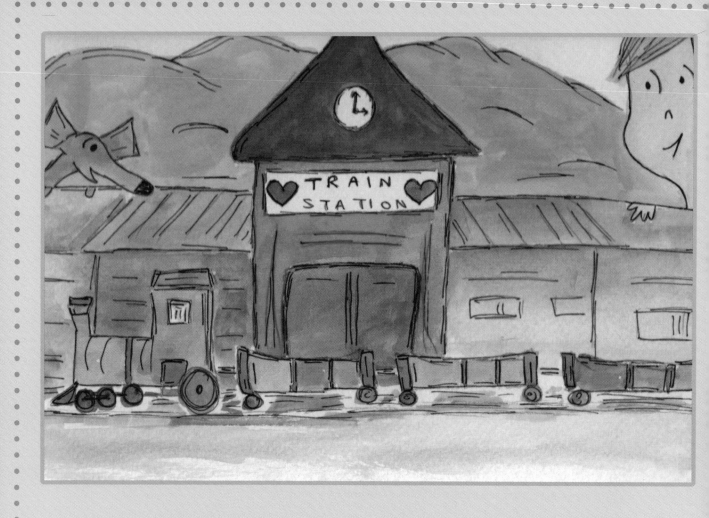

To understand, I imagine a heart as a train station.
The train and its passengers are blood flow.
The train tracks are blood vessels.
Silly, I know. But let me explain.

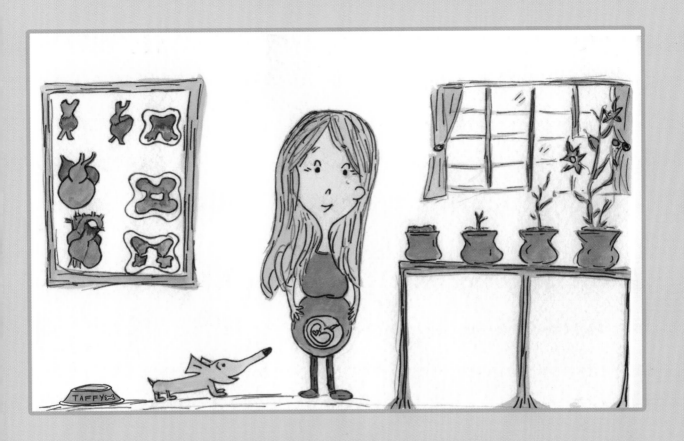

Before we are born, we begin like a small seed and the different parts of our body start to slowly form. Like our arms. Our legs. Our head and our hair. Our liver. And of course, our heart!

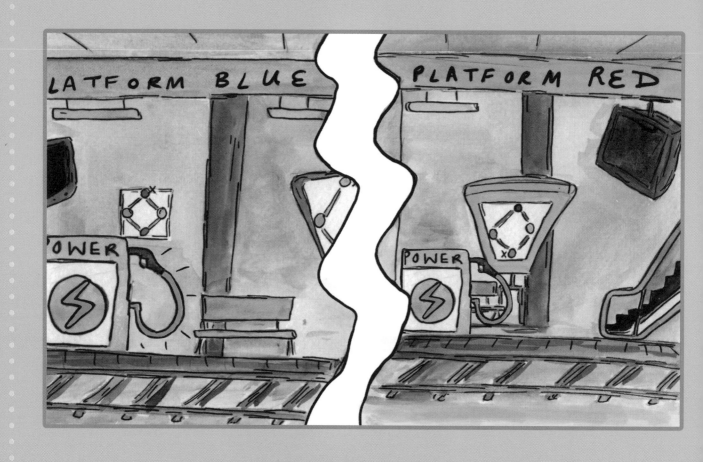

Our heart first looks like a big open tunnel —
the beginning of our train station!
As it forms, the tunnel becomes two big
train station platforms.
I call them platform BLUE and platform RED.

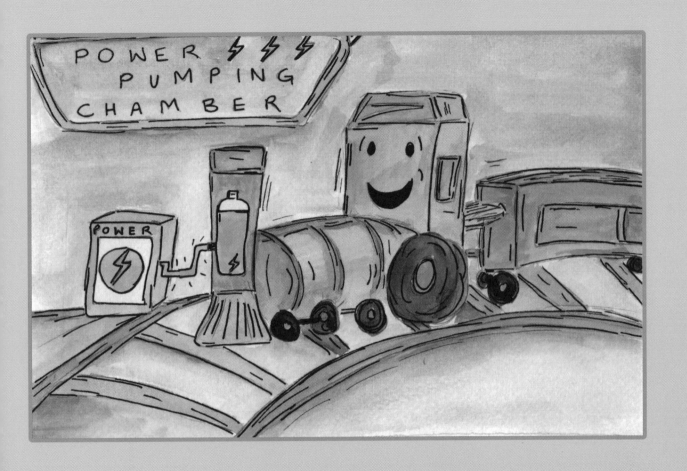

Each platform has a power pumping chamber
— our ventricle.
This is where the train gets powered up!
Just like a phone battery.

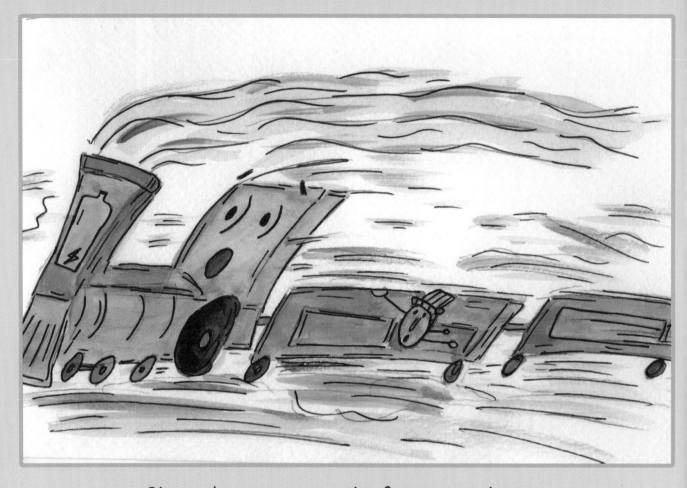

Since there are two platforms in a heart,
that means there are two power pumping stations
(two ventricles) to fire the train up at
different parts in its journey.
This power keeps the train chugging along –
full steam ahead!

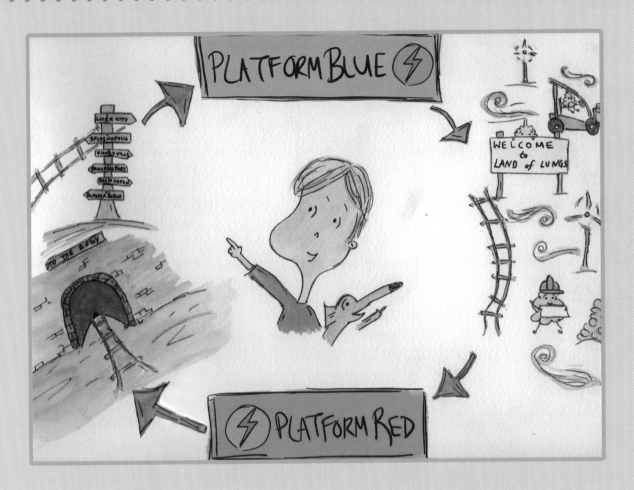

Now platform RED and platform BLUE are connected
– by train tracks — our blood vessels.
The train tracks form a huge circle around our body
so we can deliver blood everywhere.
Check out the path!

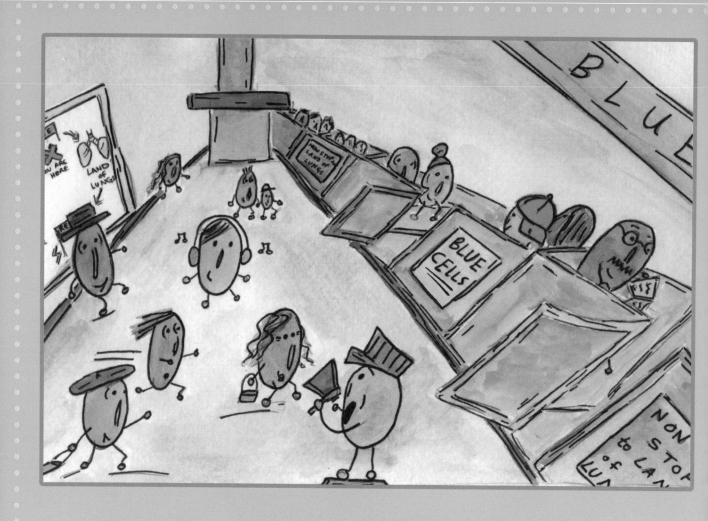

Blood cells in our body are the passengers on the train.
They come from all over.
From our head and our toes, our spleen or our nose.
Their travel on the train is the flow of blood in our body.
All aboard!

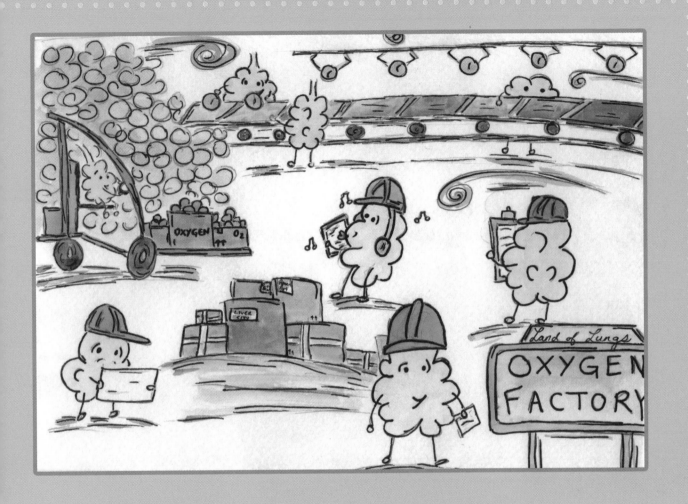

The blood cell's job is to be like a mail carrier,
delivering oxygen around your body.
You see, our bodies need oxygen to work.
When you breathe in, air – filled with oxygen –
enters your lungs.

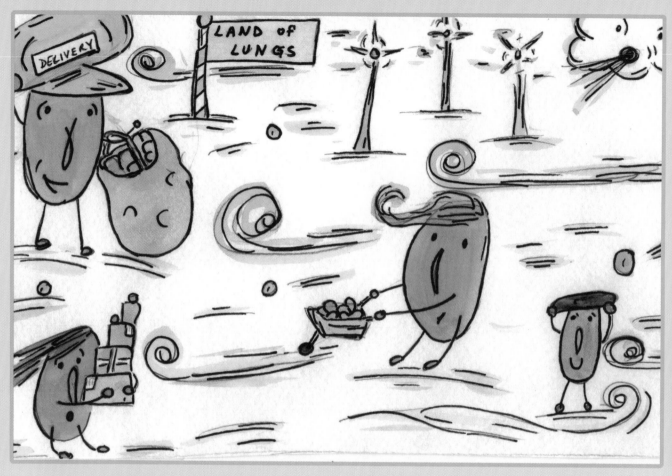

Then our blood cells pick up those
oxygen packages at the Land of Lungs.
Look how windy it is!
Hold on to your hat!

Check out how a blue cell
becomes a red cell! Just add oxygen!

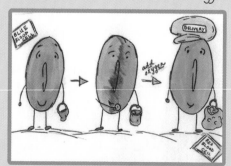

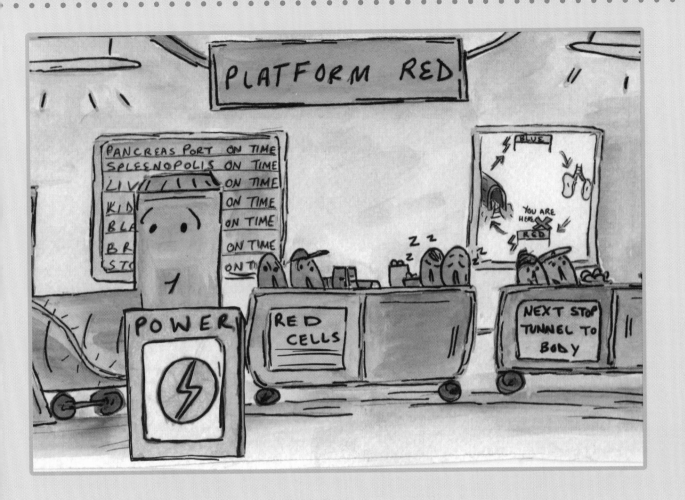

The blood cells, with their oxygen packages,
head on to the next station, Platform RED.
The train gets powered up again
and shoots out to the rest of the body.

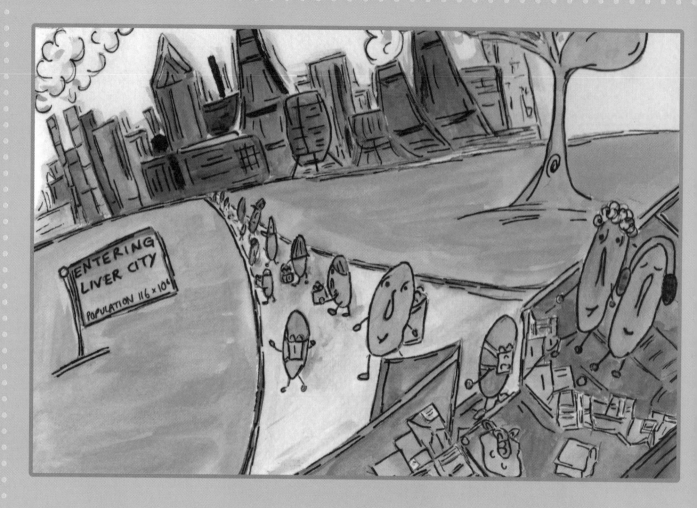

The train takes our blood cells to all sorts of cool places, like Liver City, Spleen-opolis, and Kidneyville, delivering oxygen packages wherever they go.

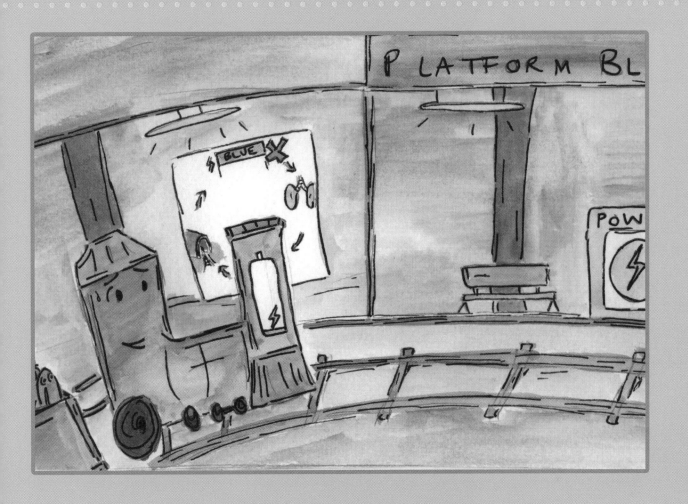

Once all the oxygen is delivered,
it's time to return to Platform BLUE.
There the train gets powered up again.
Now off to the Land of Lungs for more oxygen packages.
Let's start this journey all over again!

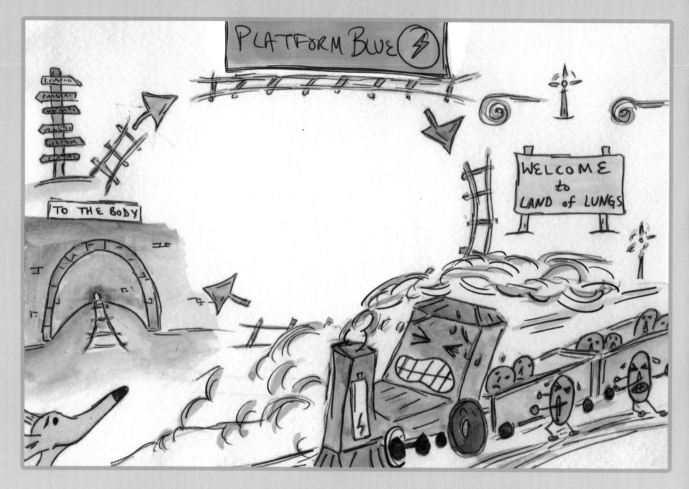

Now in single ventricle, our hearts are different.
We were born with only one power pumping chamber.
This means our train only gets powered up once for its
entire journey. One push of power to go to the
Land of Lungs, all over the body, and then return.
That's a long way to go with only one push of power.

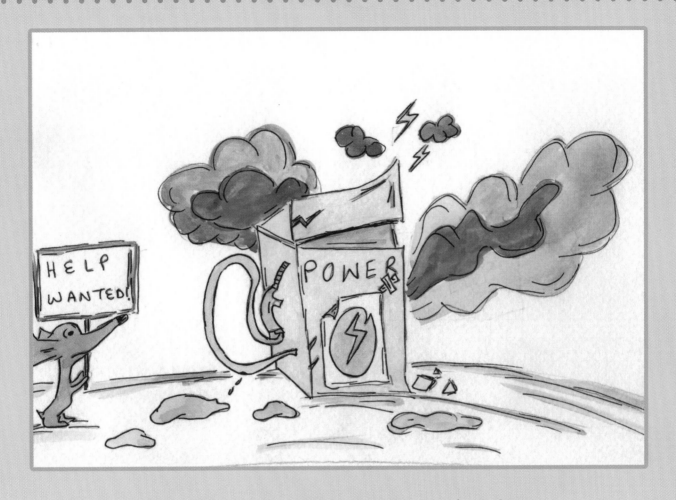

This tires our single pumping chamber.
It must do twice the work! Exhausting!
So, what can we do? How can we help our hearts?
Well first, we need to know which
power pumping chamber is missing.

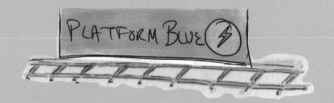

PLATFORM BLUE ⚡

If Platform BLUE's power pumping chamber is missing, our RED pumping chamber has to do all the work!
This means no power pump before our train continues to the Land of Lungs.

If Platform RED's power pumping chamber is missing, our BLUE pumping chamber has to do all the work! This means there is no power pump before the journey to the body. So it's hard for our train to travel to Liver City or Spleen-opolis.

WELCOME to LAND of LUNGS

LIVER CITY
SPLEENOPOLIS
KIDNEY VILLE
PANCREAS PORT
BRAIN HAVEN
BLADDER BEACH

TO THE BODY

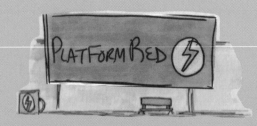

PLATFORM RED ⚡

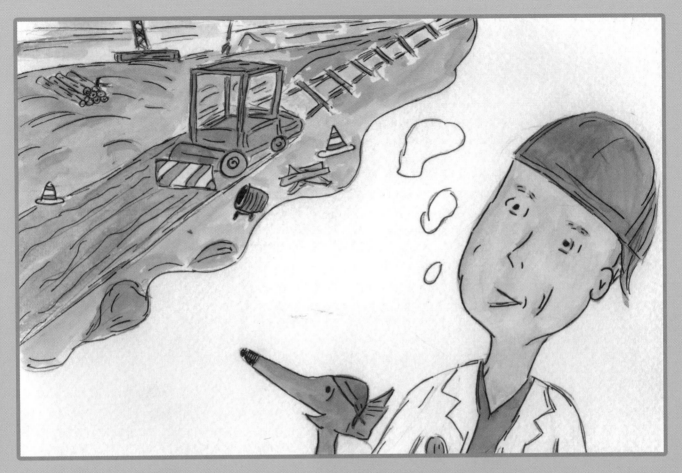

To fix this, we need three surgeries.
These surgeries are complicated, but I'll try to make it easy for you. Surgery simply rearranges your train tracks – or your blood flow. These new connections help your one power pumping chamber, so your train can make the full journey with only half the battery. Way to go!

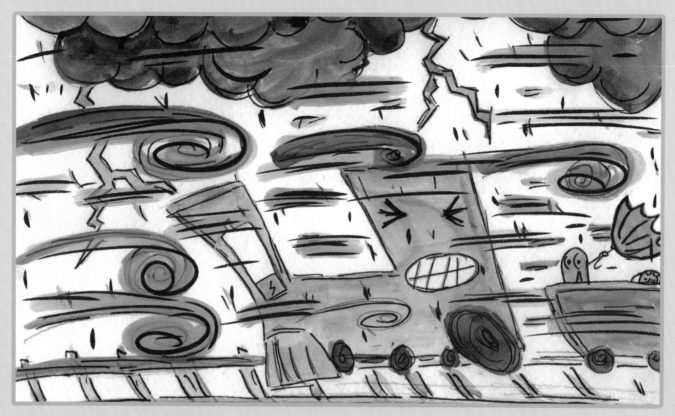

Now listen carefully. This part is important. Even after surgery, we still have only one power pumping chamber. So, we must keep it healthy and happy so our trains can keep delivering oxygen. This isn't perfect. Anything that slows down our trains can hurt us. Like getting sick. Imagine being sick is like your train trying to travel through bad weather. Without two pumping power chambers, it's harder for your train to keep chugging against terrible winds!

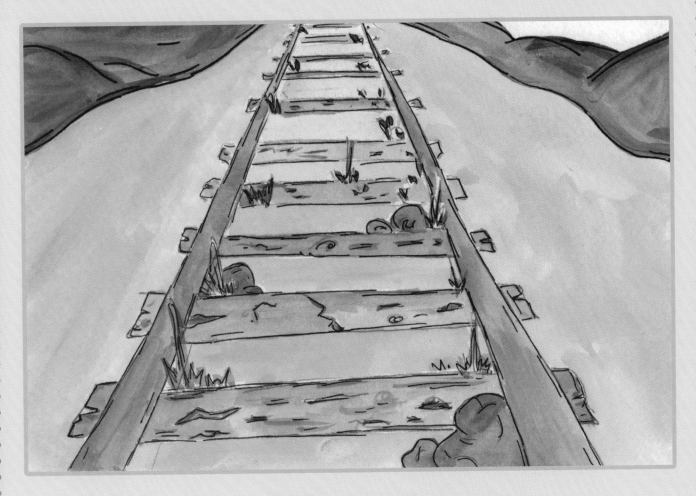

Eating a bad diet or not being active
can also hurt our train tracks.
Weeds will grow;
the tracks will narrow and break.
The more we hurt our tracks,
the harder our one power pumping chamber has to work. 21

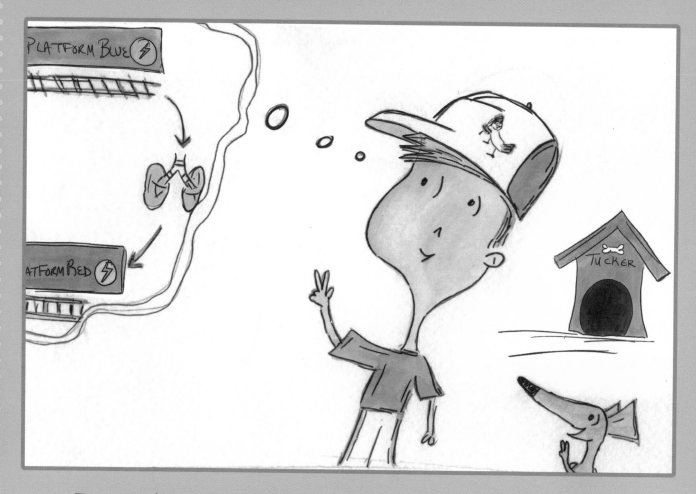

Eventually, we may need a new power pump altogether.
This means it's time for a heart transplant
— a whole new train station with TWO functioning pumps.
Can you imagine?
A new heart!

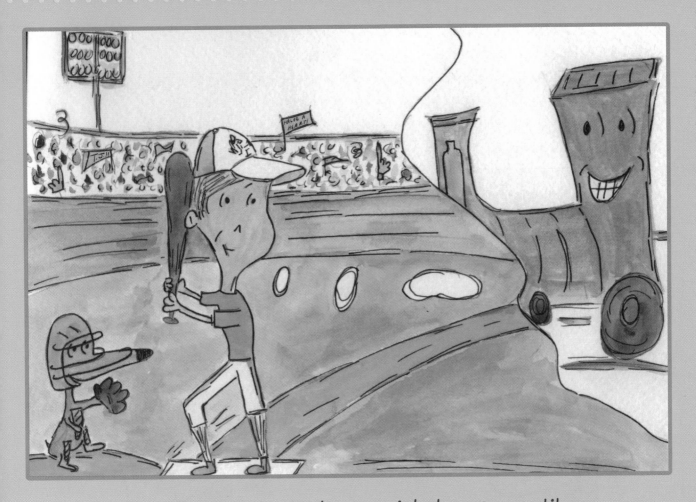

So, you see, our single ventricle hearts are like
train stations – but with only one power pump.
We only get one PUSH, or PUMP, of power
to get our blood cells everywhere.
So, let's keep our pumps happy and our trains moving!
All aboard!

A map!

Here's a map to compare
a real heart to the story's train station!

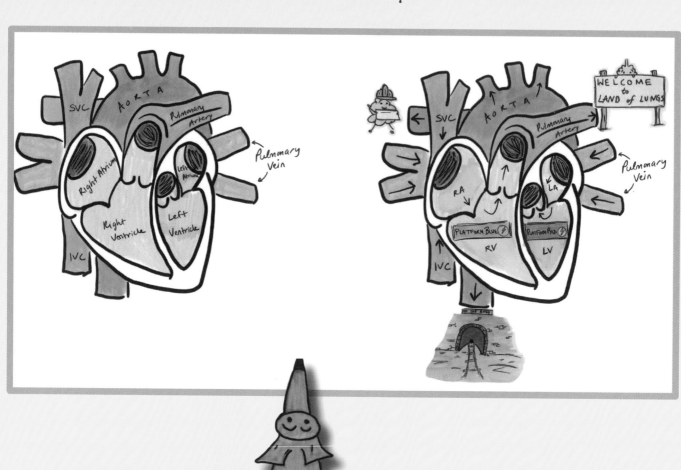

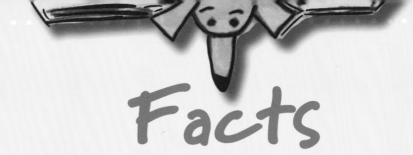

Facts

Single ventricle heart defects are when one of your ventricles (the pumping chambers in your heart) is not strong enough **or** is not big enough to do its work. This means that only one pumping chamber works – instead of typically two.

Single ventricle defects are uncommon.
They happen in 5 out of 100,000 new babies.

We usually do not know why this happens - it mostly happens by chance.

Diagnosis usually happens before birth during a prenatal ultrasound.

Most babies can have a normal delivery.

It can also be diagnosed after you are born.

A special ultrasound that is called an echocardiogram will be ordered to look at your heart.

Common signs/symptoms:
- cyanosis (looking blue)
- trouble breathing
- heart murmur (whooshing sound)

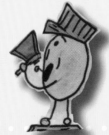

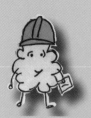

Surgery – Stage 1 Norwood or Shunt

Goal: To balance the amount of blood flowing to your lungs (a shunt procedure) and to your body (a Norwood procedure). After Stage 1, you still have one pump pumping ALL the blood to your body and lungs.

Age: 1 week old; before you go home from the hospital!

Hospital stay: Often about 1 month long (but may be longer or shorter).

Where: First, you'll stay in the ICU (usually for about a week). Then you'll move to a regular hospital bed. Your family is ALWAYS welcome! 24/7!

Your goals: To gain weight and work on feeding. You may need a tube in your nose (a nasogastric tube) or a tube in your belly (a G-tube) to help.

After you leave the hospital: You'll see your team usually every other week until your second surgery. Right before your second surgery you'll have a cardiac catheterization.

Stage 2- Glenn

Goal: This surgery helps your one pump do LESS work by making half of your blood returning to your heart, go straight to your lungs 'passively'. Imagine a train coasting downhill – it does not need any pumping power!

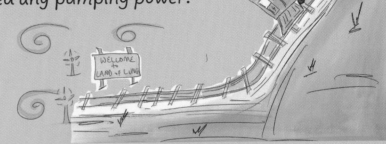

Age: 4-6 months old

Hospital stay: Usually 1-2 weeks (You'll get to see all your old friends. And yes, they do remember you!)

Where: The ICU for usually a little less than a week. Then to a regular hospital bed.

Your goals: Recovering and going back to being a typical, happy baby!

After you leave the hospital: You'll see your team usually every month to every 3 months until your third surgery. Right before your third surgery you'll have a cardiac catheterization.

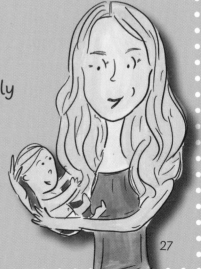

Stage 3- Fontan

Goal: This surgery also helps your one pump do LESS work by making the other half of your blood returning to your heart, go straight to your lungs 'passively'. Now all your blue blood that is returning from your body passively flows to your lungs (like coasting downhill) so your ventricle (pumping chamber) only has to do HALF the work it did before. It only has to pump blood to the body.

Age: 3 years old

Hospital stay: Usually 2 weeks

Where: The ICU for often just a couple of days. Then to a regular hospital bed.

Your goals: Recovering and getting chest tubes out.

After you leave the hospital: Your team will keep a close eye on you. You'll get labs often to keep an eye on your body – like your liver! Eventually, you may get a heart transplant. The time to needing a transplant is different for every person.

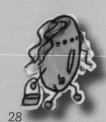

Doctor Words

Hypoplastic – not formed or underdeveloped

Chambers — a healthy heart has 4 chambers – 2 atria and 2 ventricles

Atrium – the upper chambers of the heart. There are 2 and they receive blood from the body and from the lungs.

Ventricles – the lower PUMPING chambers of the heart. There are 2. One pumps red blood to the body, the other pumps blue blood to the lungs.

Cyanosis – blue color in skin, lips or nails, which means low oxygen to your cells

Pulmonary – fancy word for lungs

Circulation— the blood flow through your blood vessels

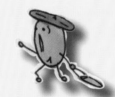

Congenital– something you are born with; not acquired

Cardiac catheterization— a tiny catheter is put into a blood vessel in your groin. It is threaded up, all the way to your heart. Dye is put into it so the heart and blood vessels can be seen. It also measures blood pressure and oxygen levels.

Echocardiogram (ECHO) – a special type of ultrasound that looks closely at the heart and measures its function. This does not hurt, and you can even watch it happen.

Electrocardiogram (EKG) – a painless test that looks at the electrical activity of the heart

Prenatal echo— an ultrasound through mom's tummy to look at your heart – how cool!

Notes

Notes

Meet the Author:
Dr. Maria Baimas-George

Maria Baimas-George MD MPH is a surgeon, training to specialize in abdominal transplantation. Inspired by her patients and mentors, she writes and illustrates books explaining medical and surgical conditions to children and their loved ones. Her goal is to create books that provide useful information to help with understanding and to offer comfort and hope.

WINNER OF THE
2021 SILVER
TOUCHSTONE
AWARD

Awarded for exceptional performance in patient safety,
clinical outcomes, efficiency & service excellence

Please visit us online at
www.StrengthOfMyScars.com to learn more about our team
and story and see our full collection of available books.

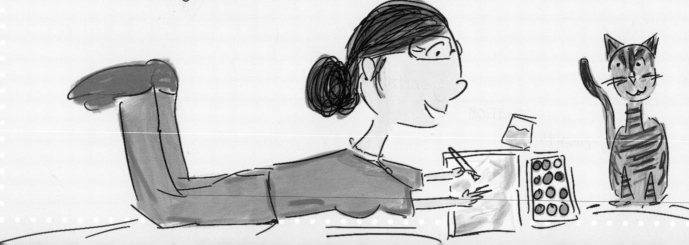